# This Journal

## FOR HOMEMADE HOUSEHOLD CLEANERS & BEAUTY PRODUCTS

## BELONGS TO

_____

_____

# Recipe for _____

| |
|---|
| TITLE |

| |
|---|
| PREP TIME |

| |
|---|
| USED FOR |

ADDITIONAL USES

NOTES

I LOVE THIS PRODUCT
BECAUSE

INGREDIENTS

# Recipe for _____

TITLE

PREP TIME

USED FOR

ADDITIONAL USES

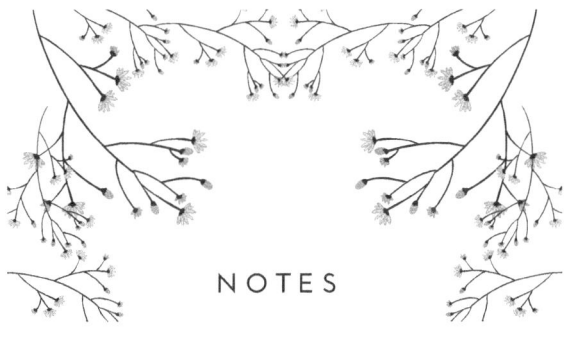

NOTES

_____

_____

_____

I LOVE THIS PRODUCT
BECAUSE

INGREDIENTS

_____

_____

_____

_____

_____

_____

_____

_____

_____

# Recipe for _____

| |
|---|
| TITLE |

| |
|---|
| PREP TIME |

| |
|---|
| USED FOR |

ADDITIONAL USES

NOTES

I LOVE THIS PRODUCT BECAUSE

INGREDIENTS

# Recipe for _____

| TITLE |
| --- |
|  |

| PREP TIME |
| --- |
|  |

| USED FOR |
| --- |
|  |

| ADDITIONAL USES |
| --- |
|  |

NOTES

I LOVE THIS PRODUCT
BECAUSE

INGREDIENTS

# Recipe for _____

| TITLE |
| --- |
| |

| PREP TIME |
| --- |
| |

| USED FOR |
| --- |
| |

| ADDITIONAL USES |
| --- |
| |

NOTES

_____

_____

_____

I LOVE THIS PRODUCT BECAUSE

INGREDIENTS

_____

_____

_____

_____

_____

_____

_____

_____

_____

# Recipe for _____

| TITLE |
|---|
|  |

| PREP TIME |
|---|
|  |

| USED FOR |
|---|
|  |

| ADDITIONAL USES |
|---|
|  |

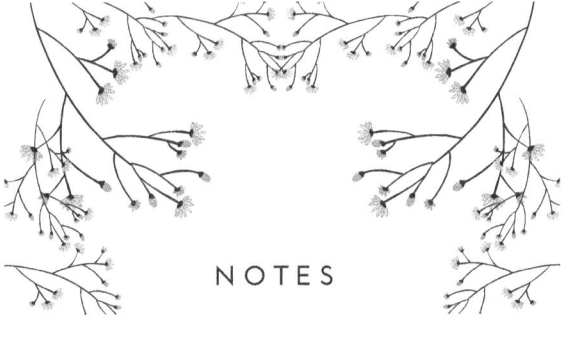

NOTES

_____

_____

_____

I LOVE THIS PRODUCT
BECAUSE

INGREDIENTS

_____

_____

_____

_____

_____

_____

_____

_____

_____

# Recipe for _____

| TITLE |
| --- |

| PREP TIME |
| --- |

| USED FOR |
| --- |

| ADDITIONAL USES |
| --- |

NOTES

I LOVE THIS PRODUCT
BECAUSE

INGREDIENTS

# Recipe for _____

| TITLE |
| --- |
| |

| PREP TIME |
| --- |
| |

| USED FOR |
| --- |
| |

| ADDITIONAL USES |
| --- |
| |

NOTES

_____

_____

_____

I LOVE THIS PRODUCT
BECAUSE

INGREDIENTS

_____

_____

_____

_____

_____

_____

_____

_____

_____

# Recipe for _____

| |
|---|
| TITLE |

| |
|---|
| PREP TIME |

| |
|---|
| USED FOR |

| |
|---|
| ADDITIONAL USES |

I LOVE THIS PRODUCT
BECAUSE

INGREDIENTS

NOTES

# Recipe for _____

| TITLE |
| --- |

| PREP TIME |
| --- |

| USED FOR |
| --- |

ADDITIONAL USES

NOTES

I LOVE THIS PRODUCT BECAUSE

INGREDIENTS

# Recipe for _____

| |
|---|
| TITLE |

| |
|---|
| PREP TIME |

| |
|---|
| USED FOR |

| |
|---|
| ADDITIONAL USES |

NOTES

_____

_____

I LOVE THIS PRODUCT
BECAUSE

INGREDIENTS

_____

_____

_____

_____

_____

_____

_____

_____

_____

_____

# Recipe for _____

| |
|---|
| TITLE |

| |
|---|
| PREP TIME |

| |
|---|
| USED FOR |

| |
|---|
| ADDITIONAL USES |

NOTES

_____

_____

_____

I LOVE THIS PRODUCT
BECAUSE

INGREDIENTS

_____

_____

_____

_____

_____

_____

_____

_____

_____

_____

# Recipe for _____

| TITLE |
| --- |

| PREP TIME |
| --- |

| USED FOR |
| --- |

| ADDITIONAL USES |
| --- |

NOTES

_____

_____

_____

I LOVE THIS PRODUCT
BECAUSE

INGREDIENTS

_____

_____

_____

_____

_____

_____

_____

_____

_____

_____

# Recipe for _____

TITLE

PREP TIME

USED FOR

ADDITIONAL USES

I LOVE THIS PRODUCT
BECAUSE

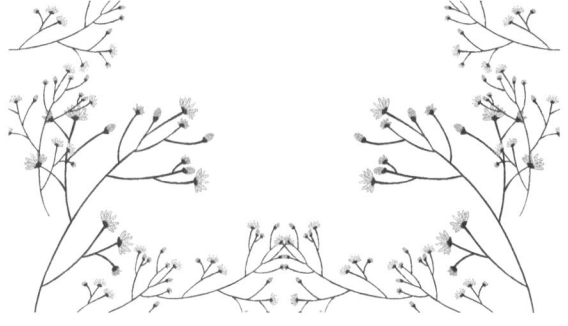

INGREDIENTS

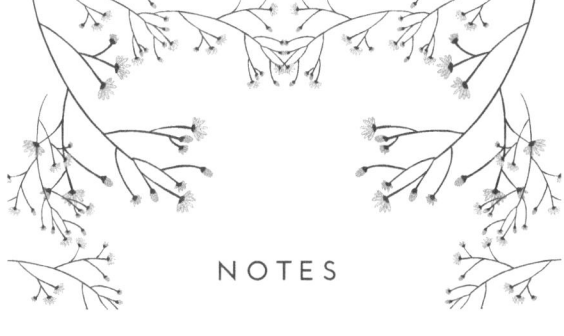

NOTES

# Recipe for _____

| TITLE |
| --- |
|  |

| PREP TIME |
| --- |
|  |

| USED FOR |
| --- |
|  |

| ADDITIONAL USES |
| --- |
|  |

NOTES

_____

_____

_____

I LOVE THIS PRODUCT
BECAUSE

INGREDIENTS

_____

_____

_____

_____

_____

_____

_____

_____

_____

_____

_____

# Recipe for _____

| TITLE |
|---|
|  |

| PREP TIME |
|---|
|  |

| USED FOR |
|---|
|  |

| ADDITIONAL USES |
|---|
|  |

NOTES

_____

_____

_____

I LOVE THIS PRODUCT
BECAUSE

INGREDIENTS

_____

_____

_____

_____

_____

_____

_____

_____

_____

# Recipe for _____

| TITLE |
| --- |

| PREP TIME |
| --- |

| USED FOR |
| --- |

| ADDITIONAL USES |
| --- |

NOTES

I LOVE THIS PRODUCT BECAUSE

INGREDIENTS

# Recipe for _____

| TITLE |
| --- |
|  |

| PREP TIME |
| --- |
|  |

| USED FOR |
| --- |
|  |

| ADDITIONAL USES |
| --- |
|  |

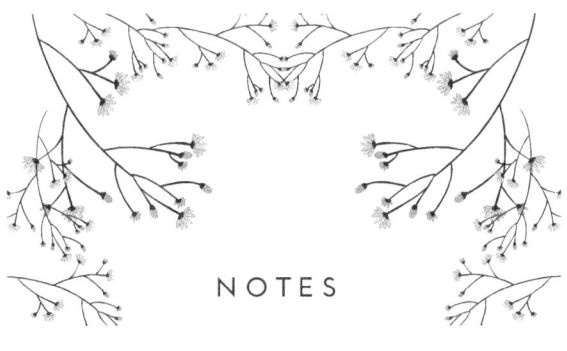

NOTES

I LOVE THIS PRODUCT
BECAUSE

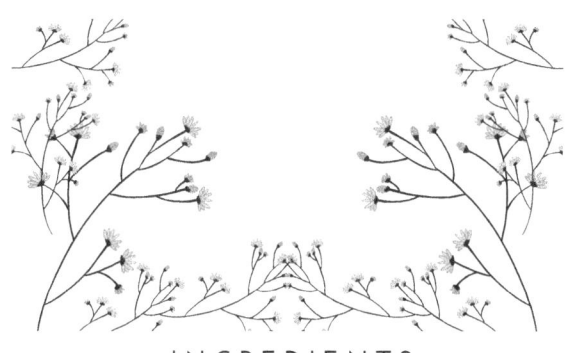

INGREDIENTS

# Recipe for _____

| |
|---|
| TITLE |

| |
|---|
| PREP TIME |

| |
|---|
| USED FOR |

| |
|---|
| ADDITIONAL USES |

NOTES

_____

_____

_____

I LOVE THIS PRODUCT
BECAUSE

INGREDIENTS

_____
_____
_____
_____
_____
_____
_____
_____

# Recipe for _____

| |
|---|
| TITLE |

| |
|---|
| PREP TIME |

| |
|---|
| USED FOR |

| |
|---|
| ADDITIONAL USES |

I LOVE THIS PRODUCT
BECAUSE

INGREDIENTS

NOTES

# Recipe for _____

| |
|---|
| TITLE |

| |
|---|
| PREP TIME |

| |
|---|
| USED FOR |

| |
|---|
| ADDITIONAL USES |

NOTES

I LOVE THIS PRODUCT BECAUSE

INGREDIENTS

# Recipe for _____

TITLE

PREP TIME

USED FOR

ADDITIONAL USES

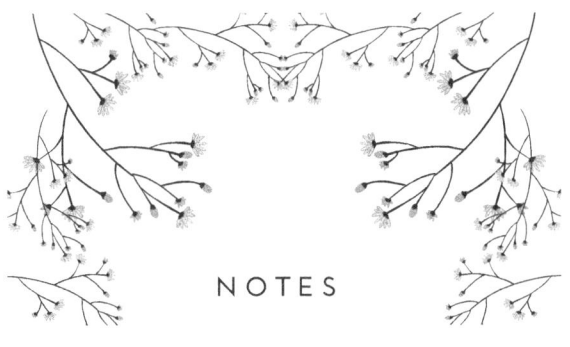

NOTES

I LOVE THIS PRODUCT
BECAUSE

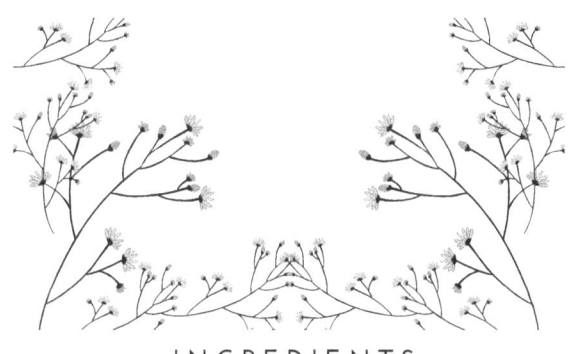

INGREDIENTS

# Recipe for _____

TITLE

PREP TIME

USED FOR

ADDITIONAL USES

NOTES

I LOVE THIS PRODUCT
BECAUSE

INGREDIENTS

# Recipe for _____

| TITLE |
| --- |
|  |

| PREP TIME |
| --- |
|  |

| USED FOR |
| --- |
|  |

| ADDITIONAL USES |
| --- |
|  |

NOTES

I LOVE THIS PRODUCT
BECAUSE

INGREDIENTS

# Recipe for _____

TITLE

PREP TIME

USED FOR

ADDITIONAL USES

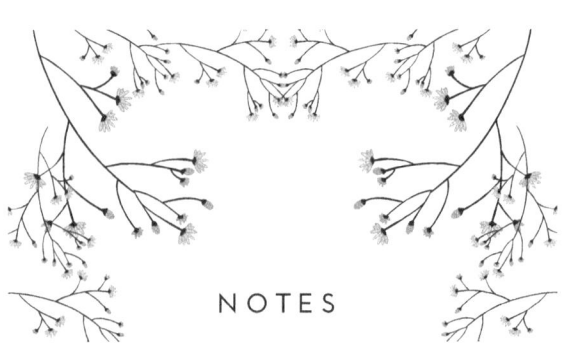

NOTES

I LOVE THIS PRODUCT
BECAUSE

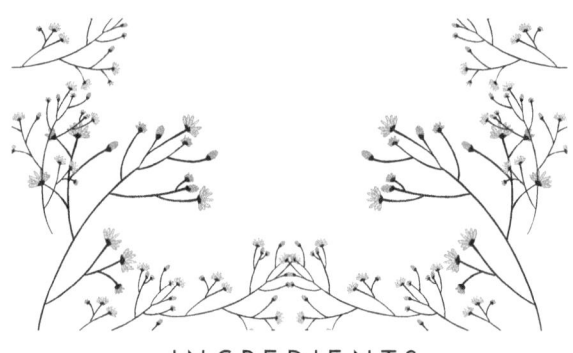

INGREDIENTS

# Recipe for _____

| |
|---|
| TITLE |

| |
|---|
| PREP TIME |

| |
|---|
| USED FOR |

| |
|---|
| ADDITIONAL USES |

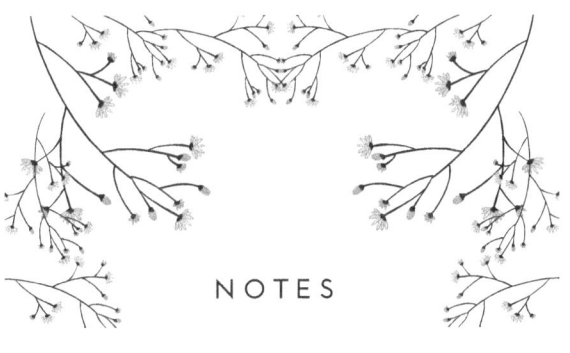

NOTES

_____

_____

_____

I LOVE THIS PRODUCT
BECAUSE

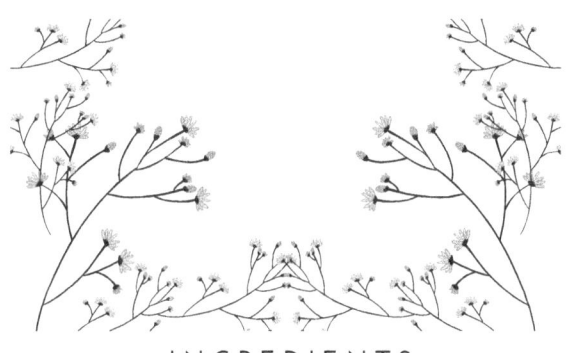

INGREDIENTS

_____

_____

_____

_____

_____

_____

_____

_____

_____

_____

# Recipe for _____

| TITLE |
| --- |
|  |

| PREP TIME |
| --- |
|  |

| USED FOR |
| --- |
|  |

| ADDITIONAL USES |
| --- |
|  |

NOTES

_____

_____

_____

I LOVE THIS PRODUCT BECAUSE

INGREDIENTS

_____

_____

_____

_____

_____

_____

_____

_____

_____

# Recipe for _____

| TITLE |
|---|
|  |

| PREP TIME |
|---|
|  |

| USED FOR |
|---|
|  |

| ADDITIONAL USES |
|---|
|  |

NOTES

_____

_____

I LOVE THIS PRODUCT
BECAUSE

INGREDIENTS

_____

_____

_____

_____

_____

_____

_____

_____

_____

# Recipe for _____

| TITLE |
|---|
| |

| PREP TIME |
|---|
| |

| USED FOR |
|---|
| |

| ADDITIONAL USES |
|---|
| |

NOTES
_____
_____
_____

I LOVE THIS PRODUCT
BECAUSE

INGREDIENTS

_____
_____
_____
_____
_____
_____
_____
_____
_____
_____
_____

# Recipe for _____

| TITLE |
| :---: |
|  |

| PREP TIME |
| :---: |
|  |

| USED FOR |
| :---: |
|  |

| ADDITIONAL USES |
| :---: |
|  |

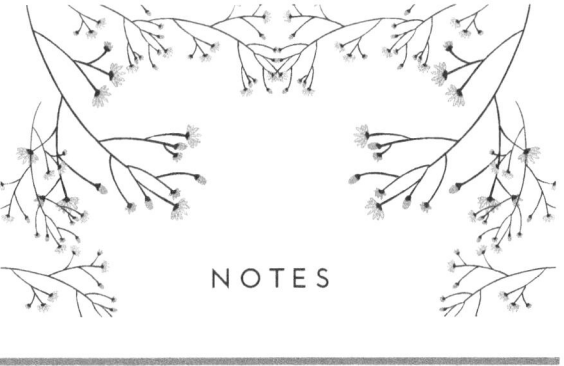

NOTES

_____

_____

_____

I LOVE THIS PRODUCT
BECAUSE

INGREDIENTS

_____

_____

_____

_____

_____

_____

_____

_____

_____

_____

# Recipe for _____

| TITLE |
|---|

| PREP TIME |
|---|

| USED FOR |
|---|

| ADDITIONAL USES |
|---|

NOTES

_____

_____

_____

I LOVE THIS PRODUCT
BECAUSE

INGREDIENTS

_____

_____

_____

_____

_____

_____

_____

_____

_____

_____

# Recipe for _____

| TITLE |
|---|
| |

| PREP TIME |
|---|
| |

| USED FOR |
|---|
| |

| ADDITIONAL USES |
|---|
| |

NOTES

I LOVE THIS PRODUCT
BECAUSE

INGREDIENTS

# Recipe for _____

| TITLE |
|---|
| |

| PREP TIME |
|---|
| |

| USED FOR |
|---|
| |

| ADDITIONAL USES |
|---|
| |

NOTES

I LOVE THIS PRODUCT
BECAUSE

INGREDIENTS

_____

_____

_____

_____

_____

_____

_____

_____

_____

# Recipe for

TITLE

PREP TIME

USED FOR

ADDITIONAL USES

I LOVE THIS PRODUCT
BECAUSE

INGREDIENTS

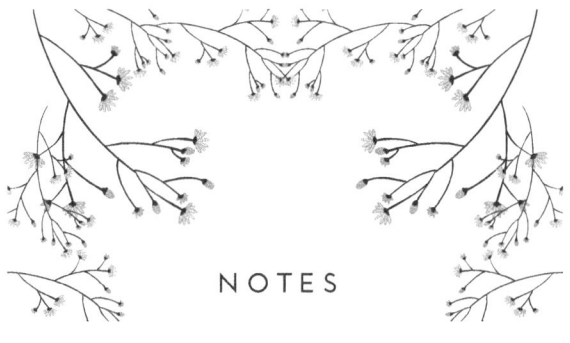

NOTES

# Recipe for _____

| TITLE |
| --- |
| |

| PREP TIME |
| --- |
| |

| USED FOR |
| --- |
| |

| ADDITIONAL USES |
| --- |
| |

NOTES

I LOVE THIS PRODUCT
BECAUSE

INGREDIENTS

# Recipe for _____

| TITLE |
|---|
|  |

| PREP TIME |
|---|
|  |

| USED FOR |
|---|
|  |

| ADDITIONAL USES |
|---|
|  |

NOTES

_____

_____

_____

I LOVE THIS PRODUCT
BECAUSE

INGREDIENTS

_____

_____

_____

_____

_____

_____

_____

_____

_____

_____

# Recipe for _____

TITLE

PREP TIME

USED FOR

ADDITIONAL USES

NOTES

I LOVE THIS PRODUCT BECAUSE

INGREDIENTS

# Recipe for _____

| TITLE |
| --- |
|  |

| PREP TIME |
| --- |
|  |

| USED FOR |
| --- |
|  |

| ADDITIONAL USES |
| --- |
|  |

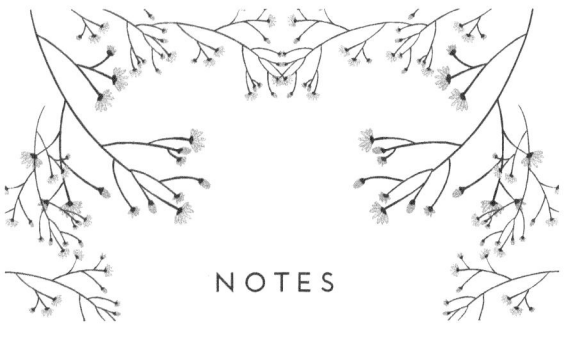

NOTES

_____

_____

_____

I LOVE THIS PRODUCT
BECAUSE

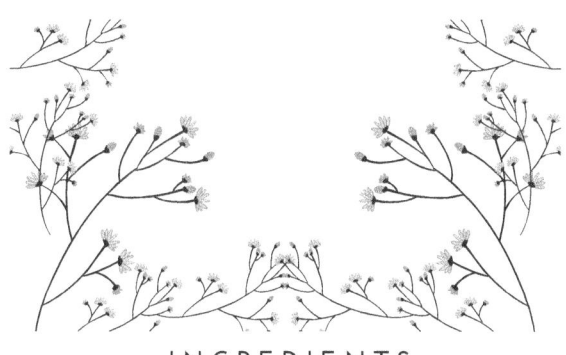

INGREDIENTS

_____

_____

_____

_____

_____

_____

_____

_____

_____

# Recipe for _____

| TITLE |
| --- |
| |

| PREP TIME |
| --- |
| |

| USED FOR |
| --- |
| |

| ADDITIONAL USES |
| --- |
| |

NOTES

I LOVE THIS PRODUCT BECAUSE

INGREDIENTS

# Recipe for _____

| TITLE |
| --- |
| |

| PREP TIME |
| --- |
| |

| USED FOR |
| --- |
| |

ADDITIONAL USES

NOTES

I LOVE THIS PRODUCT BECAUSE

INGREDIENTS

# Recipe for _____

| |
|---|
| TITLE |

| |
|---|
| PREP TIME |

| |
|---|
| USED FOR |

| |
|---|
| ADDITIONAL USES |

NOTES

_____

_____

_____

I LOVE THIS PRODUCT
BECAUSE

INGREDIENTS

_____

_____

_____

_____

_____

_____

_____

_____

_____

# Recipe for _____

| TITLE |
| --- |
| |

| PREP TIME |
| --- |
| |

| USED FOR |
| --- |
| |

| ADDITIONAL USES |
| --- |
| |

NOTES

I LOVE THIS PRODUCT BECAUSE

INGREDIENTS

# Recipe for _____

TITLE

PREP TIME

USED FOR

ADDITIONAL USES

NOTES

I LOVE THIS PRODUCT
BECAUSE

INGREDIENTS

# Recipe for _____

| TITLE |
|---|
|  |

| PREP TIME |
|---|
|  |

| USED FOR |
|---|
|  |

| ADDITIONAL USES |
|---|
|  |

NOTES

_____

_____

_____

I LOVE THIS PRODUCT BECAUSE

INGREDIENTS

_____

_____

_____

_____

_____

_____

_____

_____

_____

_____

# Recipe for _____

TITLE

PREP TIME

USED FOR

ADDITIONAL USES

NOTES

I LOVE THIS PRODUCT
BECAUSE

INGREDIENTS

# Recipe for _____

TITLE

PREP TIME

USED FOR

ADDITIONAL USES

NOTES

_____

_____

I LOVE THIS PRODUCT BECAUSE

INGREDIENTS

_____

_____

_____

_____

_____

_____

_____

_____

_____

_____

# Recipe for _____

TITLE

PREP TIME

USED FOR

ADDITIONAL USES

NOTES

I LOVE THIS PRODUCT BECAUSE

INGREDIENTS

# Recipe for _____

| TITLE |
| --- |
|  |

| PREP TIME |
| --- |
|  |

| USED FOR |
| --- |
|  |

| ADDITIONAL USES |
| --- |
|  |

NOTES

_____

_____

_____

I LOVE THIS PRODUCT BECAUSE

INGREDIENTS

_____

_____

_____

_____

_____

_____

_____

_____

_____

_____

# Recipe for _____

TITLE

PREP TIME

USED FOR

ADDITIONAL USES

NOTES

I LOVE THIS PRODUCT
BECAUSE

INGREDIENTS

# Recipe for _____

| TITLE |
| --- |
|  |

| PREP TIME |
| --- |
|  |

| USED FOR |
| --- |
|  |

| ADDITIONAL USES |
| --- |
|  |

NOTES

_____

_____

_____

I LOVE THIS PRODUCT
BECAUSE

INGREDIENTS

_____

_____

_____

_____

_____

_____

_____

_____

# Recipe for _____

TITLE

PREP TIME

USED FOR

ADDITIONAL USES

NOTES

I LOVE THIS PRODUCT BECAUSE

INGREDIENTS

# Recipe for _____

| TITLE |
|---|
|  |

| PREP TIME |
|---|
|  |

| USED FOR |
|---|
|  |

| ADDITIONAL USES |
|---|
|  |

NOTES

_____

_____

_____

I LOVE THIS PRODUCT
BECAUSE

INGREDIENTS

_____

_____

_____

_____

_____

_____

_____

_____

_____

# Recipe for _____

TITLE

PREP TIME

USED FOR

ADDITIONAL USES

NOTES

I LOVE THIS PRODUCT
BECAUSE

INGREDIENTS

# Recipe for _____

| TITLE |
| --- |

| PREP TIME |
| --- |

| USED FOR |
| --- |

ADDITIONAL USES

NOTES

I LOVE THIS PRODUCT
BECAUSE

INGREDIENTS

# Recipe for _____

TITLE

PREP TIME

USED FOR

ADDITIONAL USES

NOTES

I LOVE THIS PRODUCT
BECAUSE

INGREDIENTS

# Recipe for _____

| TITLE |
|---|
|  |

| PREP TIME |
|---|
|  |

| USED FOR |
|---|
|  |

| ADDITIONAL USES |
|---|
|  |

NOTES

_____

_____

I LOVE THIS PRODUCT
BECAUSE

INGREDIENTS

_____

_____

_____

_____

_____

_____

_____

_____

_____

# Recipe for _____

| |
|---|
| TITLE |

| |
|---|
| PREP TIME |

| |
|---|
| USED FOR |

| |
|---|
| ADDITIONAL USES |

I LOVE THIS PRODUCT
BECAUSE

INGREDIENTS

NOTES

# Recipe for _____

TITLE

PREP TIME

USED FOR

ADDITIONAL USES

NOTES

I LOVE THIS PRODUCT
BECAUSE

INGREDIENTS

# Recipe for _____

| TITLE |
| --- |
| |

| PREP TIME |
| --- |
| |

| USED FOR |
| --- |
| |

| ADDITIONAL USES |
| --- |
| |

NOTES

_____

_____

_____

I LOVE THIS PRODUCT
BECAUSE

INGREDIENTS

_____

_____

_____

_____

_____

_____

_____

_____

_____

_____

# Recipe for _____

TITLE

PREP TIME

USED FOR

ADDITIONAL USES

NOTES

I LOVE THIS PRODUCT BECAUSE

INGREDIENTS

# Recipe for _____

| TITLE |
| --- |
|  |

| PREP TIME |
| --- |
|  |

| USED FOR |
| --- |
|  |

| ADDITIONAL USES |
| --- |
|  |

NOTES

I LOVE THIS PRODUCT
BECAUSE

INGREDIENTS

# Recipe for _____

| TITLE |
| --- |
| |

| PREP TIME |
| --- |
| |

| USED FOR |
| --- |
| |

ADDITIONAL USES

I LOVE THIS PRODUCT
BECAUSE

INGREDIENTS

NOTES

# Recipe for _____

| TITLE |
|---|
|  |

| PREP TIME |
|---|
|  |

| USED FOR |
|---|
|  |

| ADDITIONAL USES |
|---|
|  |

NOTES

_____

_____

_____

I LOVE THIS PRODUCT
BECAUSE

INGREDIENTS

_____

_____

_____

_____

_____

_____

_____

_____

_____

_____

_____

# Recipe for _____

TITLE

PREP TIME

USED FOR

ADDITIONAL USES

NOTES

I LOVE THIS PRODUCT BECAUSE

INGREDIENTS

# Recipe for _____

TITLE

PREP TIME

USED FOR

ADDITIONAL USES

NOTES

I LOVE THIS PRODUCT
BECAUSE

INGREDIENTS

# Recipe for _____

| TITLE |
|---|
|  |

| PREP TIME |
|---|
|  |

| USED FOR |
|---|
|  |

| ADDITIONAL USES |
|---|
|  |

NOTES

I LOVE THIS PRODUCT
BECAUSE

INGREDIENTS

# Recipe for _____

| TITLE |
|---|
|  |

| PREP TIME |
|---|
|  |

| USED FOR |
|---|
|  |

| ADDITIONAL USES |
|---|
|  |

NOTES

_____

_____

I LOVE THIS PRODUCT
BECAUSE

INGREDIENTS

_____

_____

_____

_____

_____

_____

_____

_____

_____

# Recipe for _____

| TITLE |
|---|
| |

| PREP TIME |
|---|
| |

| USED FOR |
|---|
| |

| ADDITIONAL USES |
|---|
| |

NOTES

_____

_____

_____

I LOVE THIS PRODUCT BECAUSE

INGREDIENTS

_____

_____

_____

_____

_____

_____

_____

_____

_____

_____

# Recipe for _____

TITLE

PREP TIME

USED FOR

ADDITIONAL USES

NOTES

I LOVE THIS PRODUCT
BECAUSE

INGREDIENTS

# Recipe for _____

| | |
|---|---|
| TITLE | I LOVE THIS PRODUCT BECAUSE |
| PREP TIME | |
| USED FOR | INGREDIENTS |
| ADDITIONAL USES | |
| NOTES | |

# Recipe for _____

| TITLE |
| --- |
| |

| PREP TIME |
| --- |
| |

| USED FOR |
| --- |
| |

| ADDITIONAL USES |
| --- |
| |

NOTES

_____

_____

_____

I LOVE THIS PRODUCT
BECAUSE

INGREDIENTS

_____

_____

_____

_____

_____

_____

_____

_____

_____

# Recipe for _____

TITLE

PREP TIME

USED FOR

ADDITIONAL USES

NOTES

I LOVE THIS PRODUCT
BECAUSE

INGREDIENTS

# Recipe for _____

| TITLE |
| --- |
| |

| PREP TIME |
| --- |
| |

| USED FOR |
| --- |
| |

| ADDITIONAL USES |
| --- |
| |

NOTES

_____

_____

_____

I LOVE THIS PRODUCT
BECAUSE

INGREDIENTS

_____

_____

_____

_____

_____

_____

_____

_____

_____

_____

# Recipe for _____

| |
|---|
| TITLE |

| |
|---|
| PREP TIME |

| |
|---|
| USED FOR |

| |
|---|
| ADDITIONAL USES |

I LOVE THIS PRODUCT
BECAUSE

INGREDIENTS

NOTES

# Recipe for _____

TITLE

PREP TIME

USED FOR

ADDITIONAL USES

NOTES

I LOVE THIS PRODUCT BECAUSE

INGREDIENTS

# Recipe for _____

| TITLE |
|---|
|  |

| PREP TIME |
|---|
|  |

| USED FOR |
|---|
|  |

| ADDITIONAL USES |
|---|
|  |

NOTES

_____

_____

_____

I LOVE THIS PRODUCT
BECAUSE

INGREDIENTS

_____

_____

_____

_____

_____

_____

_____

_____

_____

# Recipe for _____

| TITLE |
| --- |

| PREP TIME |
| --- |

| USED FOR |
| --- |

| ADDITIONAL USES |
| --- |

NOTES

I LOVE THIS PRODUCT
BECAUSE

INGREDIENTS

# Recipe for _____

| TITLE |
|---|

| PREP TIME |
|---|

| USED FOR |
|---|

| ADDITIONAL USES |
|---|

NOTES
_____
_____
_____

I LOVE THIS PRODUCT
BECAUSE

INGREDIENTS

_____
_____
_____
_____
_____
_____
_____
_____
_____
_____

# Recipe for _____

| TITLE |
|---|
|  |

| PREP TIME |
|---|
|  |

| USED FOR |
|---|
|  |

| ADDITIONAL USES |
|---|
|  |

NOTES

_____

_____

_____

I LOVE THIS PRODUCT
BECAUSE

INGREDIENTS

_____

_____

_____

_____

_____

_____

_____

_____

_____

_____

# Recipe for _____

TITLE

PREP TIME

USED FOR

ADDITIONAL USES

NOTES

I LOVE THIS PRODUCT BECAUSE

INGREDIENTS

# Recipe for _____

TITLE

PREP TIME

USED FOR

ADDITIONAL USES

NOTES

I LOVE THIS PRODUCT
BECAUSE

INGREDIENTS

# Recipe for _____

TITLE

PREP TIME

USED FOR

ADDITIONAL USES

NOTES

I LOVE THIS PRODUCT
BECAUSE

INGREDIENTS

# Recipe for _____

| TITLE |
|---|
| |

| PREP TIME |
|---|
| |

| USED FOR |
|---|
| |

ADDITIONAL USES

NOTES

I LOVE THIS PRODUCT
BECAUSE

INGREDIENTS

# Recipe for _____

| TITLE |
| --- |
|  |

| PREP TIME |
| --- |
|  |

| USED FOR |
| --- |
|  |

| ADDITIONAL USES |
| --- |
|  |

NOTES

I LOVE THIS PRODUCT BECAUSE

INGREDIENTS

# Recipe for _____

TITLE

PREP TIME

USED FOR

ADDITIONAL USES

NOTES

I LOVE THIS PRODUCT
BECAUSE

INGREDIENTS

# Recipe for _____

TITLE

PREP TIME

USED FOR

ADDITIONAL USES

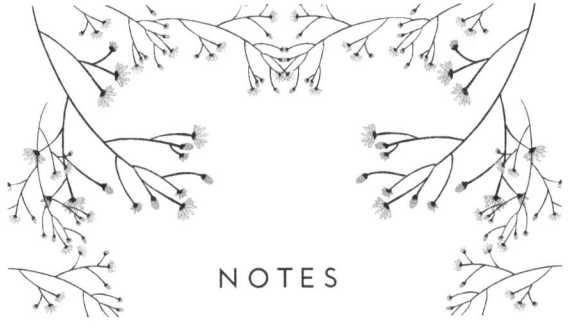

NOTES

_____

_____

_____

I LOVE THIS PRODUCT
BECAUSE

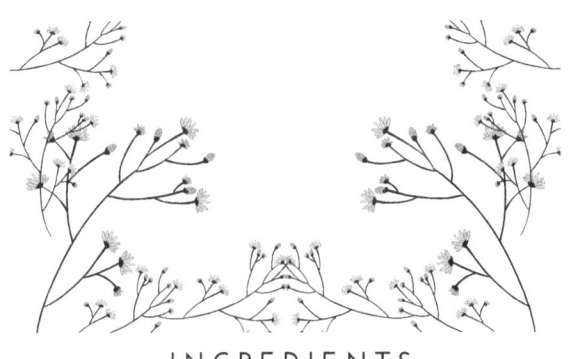

INGREDIENTS

_____

_____

_____

_____

_____

_____

_____

_____

_____

# Recipe for _____

| TITLE |
|:---:|
| |

| PREP TIME |
|:---:|
| |

| USED FOR |
|:---:|
| |

| ADDITIONAL USES |
|:---:|
| |

NOTES

_____

_____

_____

I LOVE THIS PRODUCT
BECAUSE

INGREDIENTS

_____

_____

_____

_____

_____

_____

_____

_____

_____

_____

# Recipe for _____

| TITLE |
| --- |
|  |

| PREP TIME |
| --- |
|  |

| USED FOR |
| --- |
|  |

| ADDITIONAL USES |
| --- |
|  |

NOTES

_____

_____

_____

I LOVE THIS PRODUCT
BECAUSE

INGREDIENTS

_____

_____

_____

_____

_____

_____

_____

_____

_____

# Recipe for _____

TITLE

PREP TIME

USED FOR

ADDITIONAL USES

NOTES

I LOVE THIS PRODUCT
BECAUSE

INGREDIENTS

# Recipe for _____

| TITLE |
| --- |
|  |

| PREP TIME |
| --- |
|  |

| USED FOR |
| --- |
|  |

| ADDITIONAL USES |
| --- |
|  |

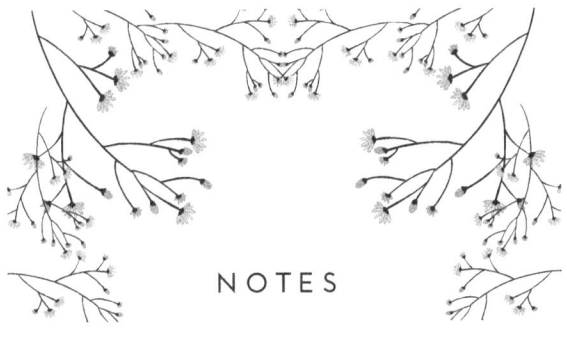

NOTES

_____

_____

_____

I LOVE THIS PRODUCT
BECAUSE

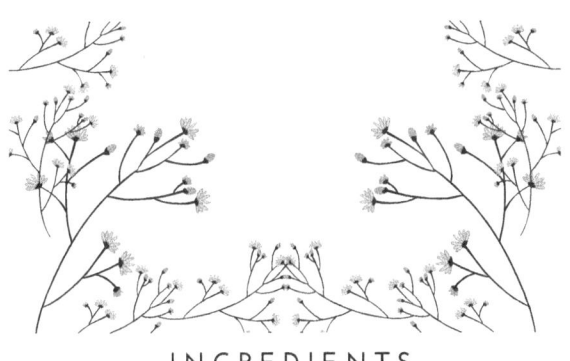

INGREDIENTS

_____

_____

_____

_____

_____

_____

_____

_____

_____

_____

# Recipe for _____

TITLE

PREP TIME

USED FOR

ADDITIONAL USES

NOTES

I LOVE THIS PRODUCT
BECAUSE

INGREDIENTS

# Recipe for _____

| TITLE |
| --- |
| |

| PREP TIME |
| --- |
| |

| USED FOR |
| --- |
| |

| ADDITIONAL USES |
| --- |
| |

NOTES

_____

_____

_____

I LOVE THIS PRODUCT BECAUSE

INGREDIENTS

_____

_____

_____

_____

_____

_____

_____

_____

_____

_____

# Recipe for _____

| TITLE |
| --- |

| PREP TIME |
| --- |

| USED FOR |
| --- |

| ADDITIONAL USES |
| --- |

NOTES

_____

_____

_____

I LOVE THIS PRODUCT
BECAUSE

INGREDIENTS

_____

_____

_____

_____

_____

_____

_____

_____

_____

_____

# Recipe for _____

TITLE

PREP TIME

USED FOR

ADDITIONAL USES

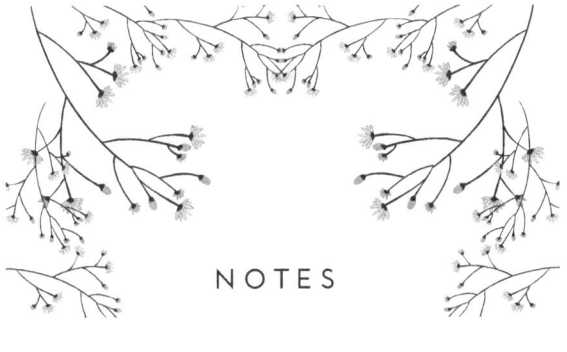

NOTES

I LOVE THIS PRODUCT
BECAUSE

INGREDIENTS

# Recipe for _____

| TITLE |
| --- |
| |

| PREP TIME |
| --- |
| |

| USED FOR |
| --- |
| |

| ADDITIONAL USES |
| --- |
| |

I LOVE THIS PRODUCT
BECAUSE

INGREDIENTS

_____

_____

_____

_____

_____

_____

_____

_____

_____

NOTES

_____

_____

# Recipe for _____

| TITLE |
| :---: |
|  |

| PREP TIME |
| :---: |
|  |

| USED FOR |
| :---: |
|  |

| ADDITIONAL USES |
| :---: |
|  |

NOTES

I LOVE THIS PRODUCT BECAUSE

INGREDIENTS

# Recipe for _____

| TITLE |
|---|
|  |

| PREP TIME |
|---|
|  |

| USED FOR |
|---|
|  |

| ADDITIONAL USES |
|---|
|  |

NOTES

_____

_____

_____

I LOVE THIS PRODUCT BECAUSE

INGREDIENTS

_____

_____

_____

_____

_____

_____

_____

_____

_____

# Recipe for _____

TITLE

PREP TIME

USED FOR

ADDITIONAL USES

NOTES

I LOVE THIS PRODUCT
BECAUSE

INGREDIENTS

# Recipe for _____

| TITLE |
| --- |

| PREP TIME |
| --- |

| USED FOR |
| --- |

| ADDITIONAL USES |
| --- |

NOTES

I LOVE THIS PRODUCT
BECAUSE

INGREDIENTS

# Recipe for _____

| TITLE |
|---|
| |

| PREP TIME |
|---|
| |

| USED FOR |
|---|
| |

| ADDITIONAL USES |
|---|
| |

NOTES

_____

_____

I LOVE THIS PRODUCT
BECAUSE

INGREDIENTS

_____

_____

_____

_____

_____

_____

_____

_____

_____

# Recipe for _____

| TITLE |
| --- |

| PREP TIME |
| --- |

| USED FOR |
| --- |

| ADDITIONAL USES |
| --- |

NOTES

I LOVE THIS PRODUCT
BECAUSE

INGREDIENTS

# Recipe for _____

| TITLE |
|---|
|  |

| PREP TIME |
|---|
|  |

| USED FOR |
|---|
|  |

| ADDITIONAL USES |
|---|
|  |

NOTES

I LOVE THIS PRODUCT
BECAUSE

INGREDIENTS

# Recipe for _____

| TITLE |
|---|
|  |

| PREP TIME |
|---|
|  |

| USED FOR |
|---|
|  |

| ADDITIONAL USES |
|---|
|  |

NOTES

_____

_____

I LOVE THIS PRODUCT
BECAUSE

INGREDIENTS

_____

_____

_____

_____

_____

_____

_____

_____

_____

# Recipe for _____

TITLE

PREP TIME

USED FOR

ADDITIONAL USES

NOTES

I LOVE THIS PRODUCT
BECAUSE

INGREDIENTS

# Recipe for _____

TITLE

PREP TIME

USED FOR

ADDITIONAL USES

NOTES

I LOVE THIS PRODUCT
BECAUSE

INGREDIENTS

# Recipe for _____

| TITLE |
|---|
| |

| PREP TIME |
|---|
| |

| USED FOR |
|---|
| |

| ADDITIONAL USES |
|---|
| |

I LOVE THIS PRODUCT
BECAUSE

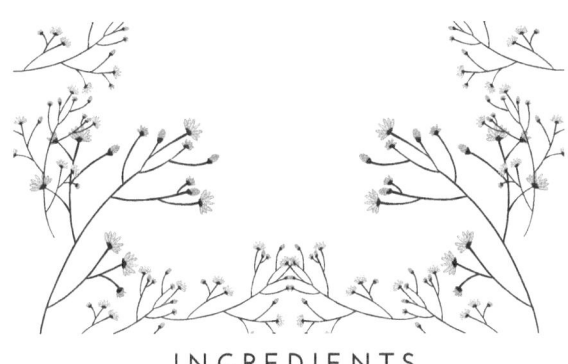

INGREDIENTS

_____

_____

_____

_____

_____

_____

_____

_____

_____

_____

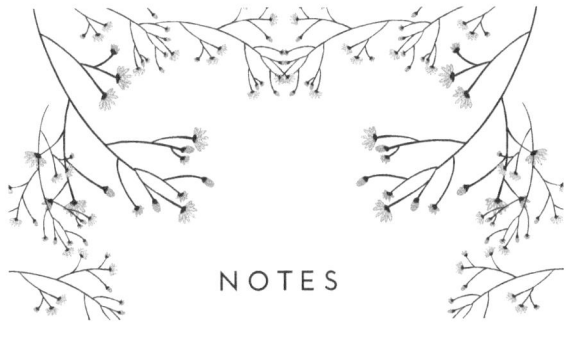

NOTES

_____

_____

# Recipe for _____

| TITLE |
| --- |

| PREP TIME |
| --- |

| USED FOR |
| --- |

| ADDITIONAL USES |
| --- |

NOTES

I LOVE THIS PRODUCT
BECAUSE

INGREDIENTS

# Recipe for _____

| TITLE |
|---|

I LOVE THIS PRODUCT
BECAUSE

| PREP TIME |
|---|

| USED FOR |
|---|

INGREDIENTS

| ADDITIONAL USES |
|---|

NOTES

# Recipe for _____

| TITLE |
| --- |

| PREP TIME |
| --- |

| USED FOR |
| --- |

| ADDITIONAL USES |
| --- |

NOTES

I LOVE THIS PRODUCT
BECAUSE

INGREDIENTS

# Recipe for _____

TITLE

PREP TIME

USED FOR

ADDITIONAL USES

I LOVE THIS PRODUCT
BECAUSE

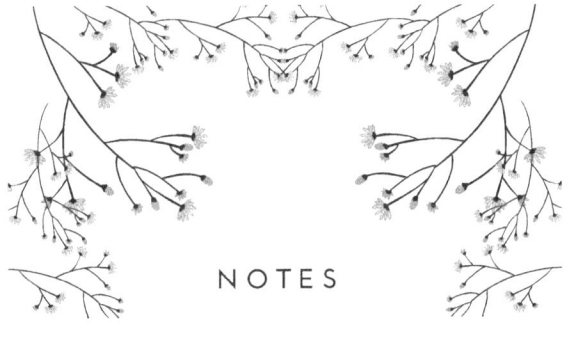

INGREDIENTS

NOTES